Weight Loss Tricks:

Tips to Escape the Dieting Trap; No Miracles, Just Facts

Charles Benson

Copyright ©2016 by CHARLES BENSON

I0423424

Table of Contents

<u>Introduction:</u>

Weight loss seems to have become more difficult as time goes by. There was a time, in the early 50's when obesity was not an issue, when no one had to worry about health related issues due to their weight and few if any people actually dieted.

Today, it seems as if everyone we come into contact with is on some type of diet, one that promises dramatic weight loss with virtually no work and yet, we are all still fat.

The dieting industry has become very rich off of promises that fail to come true, and they have also left many people feeling hopeless.

However, there is hope and throughout this book, I am going to show you exactly how to lose the weight that you have struggled with for so long. No diets, no gimmicks and no promises of a miracle, just simple facts.

<u>Chapter 1- The Truth About Weight Loss and Dieting</u>

There are so many diet techniques available, however, what we are finding is that they do not work. To start this chapter, I want to go over some of the diets that are out there and how each diet is supposed to help you lose weight.

<u>Low Carb, High Fat Diet</u>- This diet is quite

popular and it has been said to reduce the rate of heart disease. Essentially, the way that this diet works is that you will cut out all of the starchy foods that you would normally eat such as pasta, breads, potatoes, beans, fruit and rice.

Instead of eating these foods, you would instead, eat meat, eggs, fish and only plants that grow above the ground. You would also drink full fat milk, eat real butter and lard instead of seed oils.

The purpose of a low carb diet is to force a person's body to use the fat reserves for energy instead of relying on the food that is eaten. This is done by cutting out virtually all carbohydrates and eating all of the meat, fats, cheeses and butter that you want.

There are many different types of low carb, high fat diets out there, however the Atkins diet is the most popular by far.

Detox Diets- Most detox diets are very low calorie and often times the person only ingests liquids during the detoxification period. It is said that these diets will clean out the toxins from the body while ensuring that the person on the diet experiences rapid weight loss.

This is a very restrictive diet and the majority of detox diets require that you give up all of the foods that are considered toxic. Of course, these foods will vary depending on the type of detox diet that you are using. Some of them even require that you only drink water the entire time that you are on the diet.

It is said that detox diets will reset your thyroid as well as many other organs in your body in order to jump start your weight loss. Many of these diets claim that you will see as much as a 20-pound

weight loss in a short period of time as well as
clearer skin and that you will have more energy.

Slim Fast Diet- Most of us are aware of the Slim
Fast diet. According to the Slim Fast website, you
will begin by replacing breakfast and lunch with
either a shake or a nutrition bar. During the day,
you are allowed to eat 3 100 calorie Slim Fast brand
snacks followed by a dinner which can contain up
to 500 calories.

This will put your caloric intake at about 1200
calories per day and you will be getting about 100
grams of protein. Slim Fast is all about meal
replacement and controlling the amount of calories
that you eat. No one should eat less than 1200
calories per day and when a person does eat 1200
calories per day, no matter what type of calories
these are, they will lose weight, at least that is
what Slim Fast is counting on.

Slim Fast works by restricting calories as well as
what you are allowed to put into your body.
However, since there is so much protein in the

shakes, bars and snacks, the company also suggests that you do exercise regularly. This is because when you ingest a lot of protein without exercising, you will gain weight.

Paleo Diet- This diet is also known as the caveman diet because you will eat only things that were available to our ancestors during the Paleolithic age. It is said that the reason that many people are overweight is because we have more food available to us than ancient man did and that we are not supposed to be ingesting these foods.

During the Paleolithic age, people lived on what they could gather since there were no farms at the time. This means that they ate, fish, nuts, eggs, venison, poultry, roots, fruits and vegetables.

What they did not eat was dairy products, beans, peanuts, grains, potatoes or lentils. They also did not eat any processed foods and only drank water. Food was not cooked with oil and in fact most foods were not cooked at all.

A person on this diet would eat most of their foods in the raw state, however, we now know that raw

meat can make us very sick so the cooking of meat
is acceptable.

It is said that this diet is great for those that suffer
from heart disease as well as diabetes. It is claimed
that the Paleo diet makes you lose weight because
it forces your body to use the stored fat for energy
and that once you are at your ideal body weight,
you will simply stop losing weight.

According to claims by those that created the Paleo
diet, by eating the foods that are allowed, you will
level out your blood sugar, balance your hormone
production, feel more satisfied and have more
productive workouts.

Low Calorie Diet- Most people who have ever been
on a diet have been on a low calorie diet. The idea
behind a low calorie diet is to create a calorie
deficient, basically eating less calories than you
burn, but instead of burning more calories, the
dieter simply eats less in hopes that it will cause
their body to use the stored fat for energy.

A low calorie diet is one that allows less than 1200
calories per day to be eaten and most of the foods

that are allowed are low calorie, no calorie or low
fat foods.

It is important to know that there are 3500 calories
in each pound. Therefore, those that are taking
part in a low calorie diet are trying to restrict their
calories to the point of forcing their bodies to lose
a certain amount of pounds per week.

For example, if you wanted to lose 2 pounds per
week, you would need to cut 7000 calories out of
your diet each week or 1000 calories per day. If you
are only eating 1800 calories per day to begin with,
cutting 1000 out would leave you with 800 calories
per day for all of your meals.

Cutting your calories is going to make you lose
some weight, we will talk about the other effects of
a diet like this later on in this book, but it is
important to understand, a low calorie diet is a
very low energy diet.

3-hour diet- The 3-hour diet is one that can
sound as if it would be completely healthy and
actually work but let's take a look. According to
Good House Keeping, when you are on the 3-hour

diet, you will eat every three hours that you are awake.

It is also required that in order to give your metabolism a kick start in the morning; you need to eat at least 1 hour after you wake up. So a normal day would look like this:

5am- Get up, 6am- eat breakfast- 9am snack- 12- lunch- 3pm snack-6pm dinner, 9pm desert.

Each meal is supposed to contain 400 calories, each snack 100 calories and desert should contain no more than 100 calories. This is providing your body with 1500 calories per day.

This diet claims to promote weight loss over time, and claims that by never letting your body get hungry, you are ensuring that it does not go into starvation mode, which causes your metabolism to slow down and your body to hold on to fat. This diet also claims to give you 2 pounds of weight loss a week, no exercise needed.

Of course, there are hundreds, if not thousands of different diets out there that we could talk about all day long, however, I am sure that you want to

get to what really works. That's right, none of the
diets that you have read about thus far or that you
will find on the internet are going to work because,
after all, they are all just diets.

The truth is that diets simply do not work. In the
following chapter, we will look at exactly why diets
do not work, however, it is important for you to
understand that instead of working, diets are going
to trap you in an endless cycle.

You see, the diet industry is booming. If diets really
worked, they would do what they claim, cause
people to lose weight, we would move on with our
lives and never look back again.

However, what really happens is that a person goes
on a diet, works hard to follow the diet and loses a
bit of weight. Then when a person goes off of the
diet, they regain the weight and often gain more
than they lost in the first place.

A study was done in 1959 that showed 95 percent
of people who go on a diet regain the weight within
the first year of going off of the diet. These
numbers have not changed in almost 60 years,

which can lead many people to ask, why are we still dieting.

It can also make many people feel as if there is no hope, that they are going to forever be caught in this cycle of dieting and weight gain. However, there is hope and I want to teach you exactly how you can lose weight in the rest of this book.

Chapter 2- Why Regimented Diets Don't Work

There are many reasons why diets don't work and that is what I want to talk about in this chapter.

Let's first take a look at the very popular low calorie diet. This is a diet that so many people try and it is one that leads them to getting stuck in the cycle of dieting.

A low calorie diet as discussed in the previous chapter is one that is quite restrictive when it comes to calories. It is said that this diet will cause a person to lose weight because they create a calorie deficit.

When looking at this diet in the short term, yes, you may lose a few pounds, however, this diet is going to be one that is very difficult to stick to because, since you are not eating the recommended amount of calories each day, you are going to become very tired and sluggish.

The next thing that is going to happen is that you are actually going to cause your metabolism to slow down. You see, your body was created to store fat when food was scarce. This means that when your body is not getting the amount of calories that it needs, it is going to think that there is a famine and it needs to hold on to as much fat as it can.

This is going to cause you to struggle to lose the weight that you want to lose, however it is possible. But, what happens when you go off of the diet?

After you have lost the weight and you go back to eating like a normal person, your body is going to start preparing for the next time that there is a famine. Your metabolism will already be slowed down and your body will naturally begin to store the food that you eat as fat on your body simply preparing for the next time you do not feed it properly.

This is where the cycle begins. Of course, you will gain weight and find yourself on another diet in hopes of losing the weight once again.

This of course is just one example of a diet and why it does not work. However, there are many diets and many reasons that they do not work but instead force you into this dieting cycle.

One of the reasons that diets do not work is that diets actually cause our body to slow down when it comes to weight loss. The reason for this is because dieting is stressful. When our bodies are stressed, they produce a hormone called cortisol, otherwise known as the stress hormone.

This hormone causes our metabolic rate to slow down, thus causing us to burn fewer calories. It is also known for causing the body to store fat around the midsection.

The second reason why diets do not work is because they are impossible to sustain over a long period of time. You see, while you may be able to stick to a diet for a few weeks or even a few months, you are not making changes that are going to last a lifetime.

When you finish dieting, you will go back to eating normal foods again, when this happens, you will regain the weight that you lost. A diet does not get down to the root of our behaviors when it comes to food, but instead it provides us with a temporary solution.

The next reason that diets do not work is simply because they are not enjoyable. No matter what diet you are on, there is always a list of foods that you cannot eat which can make a person feel deprived. There is no pleasure when it comes to dieting which often means that here is no joy.

Instead, we become tense around food which of course raises our stress levels and we already talked about what stress can do to the body. Often times, when a person is on a diet, they do not enjoy the food that they are eating. In fact, many times, they are struggling to get through the meals no matter how hungry their body says they are and this can lead to huge cravings.

Many diets cut out complete food groups or they have you jumping in so quickly that there is no way for you to do anything but fail. It is important for you to know that the more restrictive a diet is, the less chance you have at succeeding with it.

A diet is all about willpower, not about eating what is good for you and making long term changes in your life. Instead, it is about fighting against your own body, essentially trying to demand that it does what you request of it.

Most diets also focus on calories in versus calories burned, which is a very outdated way of thinking and has been proven wrong. You see, even if you are eating 1200 calories of prepackaged diet foods such as 100 calorie snack packs, and burning tons of calories each day, you are not going to really lose the fat on your body. These foods are not really food. This type of diet food is not healthy and it is not going to help you lose weight. It is a way for companies to make money and keeps their customers dieting and coming back for more.

Finally, the main reason that diets do not work is because they make losing weight so much more complicated than it has to be.

Did you know that at least 62 percent of Americans are considered overweight or obese? It would seem that with all of the so called diets on the market, at least if these diets worked, these numbers would be much smaller.

A recent study showed that at any given time, at least 50 percent of women are on a diet, 90 percent of teenager's diet on a regular basis and as many as 50 percent of children have dieted at some point in their life.

In a survey that was conducted, it was found that almost 50 million dollars are being spent each year on dieting products in the United States alone and it is expected that those numbers are going to continue to grow.

The fact is, that when you go on a diet, the odds are really stacked against you. As I mentioned earlier, at least 95 percent of people who do lose weight on a diet gain all of the weight back within 1 year. Of those that do try and diet, 85 percent of them fail.

Let's look at it like this. If 1000 people decided to go on a diet, only 150 of them would be successful. Out of that 150, only 8 of them would be able to keep the weight off for more than 1 year. That is not a very good success rate when you think about how many people are actually starting diets each year.

However, there is hope. You have to understand that real weight loss does not come in the form of shakes, meal replacements or starvation. Instead, it comes from a healthy lifestyle.

Chapter 3- Diets to Promote Weight Loss

I hate to use the word diet because if you want to lose weight, you need to stay as far away from traditional diets as possible. Instead, I think it is important for you to understand that what I am going to talk about in this chapter is not a diet at all but it is a lifestyle change.

If you want to lose weight and keep it off, you have to make lifestyle changes. You have to get down to the basics, understand what is going on with you and the food that you eat and choose to make a change that will stick for the rest of your life.

Now, these changes are not going to happen overnight. However, by making small changes in your day to day life, in the long term, you will see huge results.

The first thing that you will want to do is to take out a notebook and start recording what you are eating every single day. You see, many people do not realize the amount of food that they are eating each day. These people often can be heard saying that they do not understand why they are not losing weight because they barely eat anything.

Remember, you can gain weight by eating too much and you can completely stop weight loss by not eating enough. Therefore, it is important for you to know exactly how many calories you are putting into your body.

The next thing that you want to look at is what you are putting in your body. While no food should ever be off limits when you are making a lifestyle change to lose weight, there should be limits set.

For example, while it is perfectly okay to grab a cheeseburger every now and then, this should not be your go to lunch on a daily basis. Instead, you should focus on getting healthy foods into your diet.

So what types of foods should you eat? You should begin by changing the way that you look at food. Real food is what comes from the earth. Fruits, vegetables, meat, dairy, grains and legumes.

Processed 'foods' are not really fuel for your body. This 'food' that should be considered junk is what many people are living off of and it is not providing their bodies with the nutrients that it needs.

Your body has to have natural foods if it is going to function properly. However, the diet industry has told us all of our lives that we should eat the low calorie, no calorie or low fat foods that they make for us in a lab instead of the foods that are made from the earth.

The good news is that when you are eating these healthy foods, you really don't have to worry too much about counting your calories. However, you should not eat until you feel as if you are going to explode.

Let's start by talking about whole grains. It is recommended that adults eat 3 to 5 servings of whole grains each day. Most people eat what is known as refined grains or white flour which has been stripped of all of its nutrients. Barley, brown rice, oats, and quinoa are all great whole grains that you can add to your diet.

Whole grains are going to help to stabilize your insulin levels, which is vital to weight loss. On top of this, they are going to provide your body with lots of vitamins and minerals that you are probably lacking in right now.

The next food you need to focus on getting in your diet are fruits and vegetables. You need to make sure that you are eating at least 2 servings of fruit each day and 3 servings of vegetables. This literally means that you need 2 cups of fruit each day and three cups of vegetables. However, when it comes to leafy greens, you will need to eat 2 cups in order to reach your one serving. One thing that many people become confused with is juice. Fruit and vegetable juice is not considered a serving of fruits or vegetables.

Juice should be limited if drank at all because when you juice fruits and vegetables, you are missing out on all of the fiber that you would get if you actually eat the fruit or vegetable as well as many other nutrients. The truth is, juice is packed full of calories and sugar, but provides you with very little nutritional value.

The next food that you want to add into your diet is legumes. These are beans, peas and peanuts. You will want to eat at least 3 servings of legumes each day, each serving being about ½ a cup

When it comes to meat, most people are eating far too much. You should only eat about 3 to 6 ounces of meat each day. This meat should be fish, poultry or other lean meat.

Dairy products such as milk, butter and cheese should be eaten every day as well, but you should only eat about 2 servings of dairy each day. This is another food that so many people are eating far too much of and no matter how healthy a food is for you, if you eat too much of it, you will gain weight and you can become sick.

You should eat no more than 2 servings of fat each day. This includes oils, mayo, butter, and salad dressing.

Sweets and anything containing added sugar should be avoided as it provides no nutritional value and will only make you fat. However, if you are craving one of your favorite foods and simply cannot say no. Take very small bits. Focusing on the flavor and once you are satisfied, put the food away instead of eating it all in one gulp.

What about drinks? Many people do not realize how much sugar and calories they are ingesting through their drinks alone. Let's look at one can of soda for example. There are about 140 calories in one can of soda, and 16 tablespoons of sugar, not to mention all of the chemicals that it contains.

Not only does sugar increase your chance of developing heart disease, but it actually increases your chance of obesity. Sugar is found in most drinks, including teas, coffee and juice. For this reason, you need to stick to drinking water.

If water is not something that you really enjoy, consider adding a few slices of lemon to your water to give it some flavor. Teas can be added to the diet if they are sweetened with honey, but again this should be only in moderation.

Many people believe that drinking a diet drink or a zero calorie drink is better than for their health than the full calorie alternative, however, there is more to a diet drink than just saving 140 calories.

Artificial sweeteners are much sweeter than sugar and studies have shown that they actually have the same effect on your body as sugar does. You see, when you drink diet drinks that are sweetened with artificial sweeteners, the insulin spikes just as it would when you drink something that contains sugar. This is because the artificial sweetener tricks your body into thinking that you are ingesting sugar. This causes your body to go into fat storage mode essentially making you gain weight.

Let's be honest, how many overweight people have you seen drinking diet soda? The fact is that we have been lead to believe that by drinking diet soda we will lose weight, however; the truth is that it can actually lead to weight gain. One study showed that those who drank diet drinks had a 70 percent more chance of gaining weight than those that did not. It was also shown that by drinking 'diet' drinks, a person increased their chances of developing metabolic syndrome by 36 percent, cholesterol levels were increased, blood pressure was

elevated, and they were at a higher chance for
having a stroke.

Diet drinks have no nutritional value whatsoever
and are made up of chemicals, not natural
ingredients. The fact is, if you want to be healthy
and lose weight, you need to drink water and avoid
anything that is packed full of sugar or artificial
sweeteners.

While there are some factors that affect a person's
metabolism that cannot be changed, when you eat
the right foods, you are going to increase your
metabolism, thus allowing you to lose more weight
in a shorter amount of time.

If you want to boost your metabolism, you can
start by eating smaller meals more frequently. For
example, instead of eating 3 meals a day, consider
eating 6 smaller meals throughout the day. This will
ensure that your metabolism does not drop in
between meals, but that your metabolic rate
remains level throughout the entire day. This will
cause you to lose more weight and have more
energy.

You want to start your day out with a healthy breakfast. Breakfast is going to jump start your metabolic rate and many studies have proven that those who eat a well-balanced breakfast are not only healthier than those that skip breakfast all together but they weigh less.

Drinking water is also very important to your metabolic rate. You see, when the body is dehydrated, the metabolism slows down and your body temperature drops. In order to keep warm, your body will begin to store fat. When you are hydrated, the water will help to flush fat from the body on the other hand, if you are dehydrated, your body will store as much fat as it can.

What about the foods that you should eat? When it comes to changing your diet and eating real food instead of processed foods, many people simply do not understand why real food is so important. After all, according to the nutritional facts, they can get all the same nutrients from processed foods.

However, you have to look at how much energy is needed to digest certain foods. When you eat a meal containing protein, fruits, and vegetables, you are going to boost your metabolism and you are going to find that your body has to work harder to digest these foods as compared to let's say a fast food cheeseburger.

This means that as the body works to digest the food, it is actually going to burn more calories where as if you were to eat the cheeseburger, the body would quickly digest it and would store it as fat.

So what does all of this mean? Your metabolic rate is determined by the number of calories it takes your body just to function each day. If you have a slow metabolism, you are not going to be able to eat the same amount of calories as someone with a high metabolism.

When this happens, you will find that eating even a small amount of calories can cause you to gain weight.

I stated earlier in this book that diets which are all or nothing do not work so how are you supposed to make these changes?

If you want to see long term weight loss that is going to be sustainable over time, you have to start out by making small changes. If you make huge changes too quickly, you will find that you cannot stick to them and no matter what you do, you will be dieting instead of making lifestyle changes.

Begin by replacing your soda, tea or juices with water, ensuring that you are drinking at least 64 ounces of water every day. As you begin to hydrate your body, you will begin to become more energetic and you will be ready to make more changes.

Next, start adding in healthy fruits and vegetables to your diet. Of course, you are going to have to cut some of the foods out that you already eat otherwise, you will just be adding more calories into a diet that is far too high in calories to begin with.

So instead of having that bag of chips while you are on break, grab an apple or some carrots with hummus. Instead of eating that baked potato with your dinner, replace it with a baked sweet potato or a side salad.

Making these small changes will add up over time and as you continue with the process, you are going to find that you are eating more of the healthy foods that your body needs and a lot less of the processed junk that it does not need.

In fact, in only a few months, you will find that the majority of your diet is going to be healthy fruits, vegetables, meats, whole grains and legumes.

By slowly replacing the foods that you are currently eating, you will not have to worry about cravings because your body is not going to miss the foods you are cutting out. However, if you were to dump all of your food in the trash, then go out and purchase only healthy foods, you would likely send your body into shock and the cravings for processed junk would hit hard.

This type of lifestyle change is not going to be a quick fix to your weight issues, and that is why many people get stuck in the cycle of dieting, however, it is going to provide you with sustainable results and you are going to feel better and be healthier than you have ever been before.

Weight Loss Tricks: Tips to Escape the Dieting Trap; No Miracles, Just Facts

Chapter 4- Need for Exercise

Anyone that has ever been on a diet knows that they are supposed to exercise, they know that if they want to be healthy, they have to exercise and that it is necessary for weight loss.

However, there are some benefits that many people do not know about. The first benefit of exercising is improvement in memory. We've all been there, we were supposed to remember something important and it completely slips our mind. We wonder what we can do in order to help us remember and after trying every gimmick on the market find there really is nothing that can be done. However, by exercising every day, we can improve our memory naturally.

Exercise also helps to improve posture. When it comes to the way that you hold your body, knowing that having bad posture can make you look much larger than you really are is very important. If you practice good posture on the other hand, you will look much thinner and appear more confident. Exercise helps to strengthen the muscles in the back, which naturally causes us to practice good posture.

I talked earlier in this book about the effects of stress on the body and how it can cause you to gain weight. What I did not mention is how you can help rid yourself of this stress. No, I am not talking about quitting your job and spending your days on the beach. I am talking about exercise. Not only does exercise release endorphins which are natural stress fighters, but it allows us to take our mind off of the things which are stressing us and just live in the moment.

Getting enough sleep is vital if you want to lose weight, however many people suffer from insomnia and it seems that no matter what they try, they cannot fall asleep. If you are having a hard time falling asleep at night, chances are you are not getting enough exercise. Whenever anyone comes to me and tells me that they cannot sleep, the first thing that I ask them is how much exercise they are getting each day. The majority of them tell me almost none.

It may seem completely opposite than what you would think would happen, but studies have shown that when you exercise, you have more energy to get you through your day. One study showed that those who exercised in the middle of the day were more productive and had more energy throughout the rest of the day and slept better at night.

When you look at all of the benefits of exercise, the truth is that by exercising, you will be a happier and healthier you. However, this is not enough to get most people to exercise.

As far as weight loss goes, we have already talked about how you have to burn more calories than you ingest. While it is true that every calorie is not equal, exercise is still important because it helps to build muscle in the body which helps to boost the metabolism which causes weight loss.

I find that it is important to explain to you, that you are in no way going to burn off the food that you eat by exercising. This is why you need to make sure that you are not overeating, or ingesting more calories than your body needs on any given day.

However, exercising does help to burn more calories and it helps to build muscle.

Let's look at it like this, let's say that you were eating 2500 calories per day and you cut back to 1500. You are now eating 1000 calories less per day than what you were but your body only needs 1500 calories per day. Therefore, simply by changing what you eat and ingesting less calories, you will not lose weight. However, by adding in exercise, let's say burning 500 calories per day, you have now created a deficit, and will lose an average of about 1 pound per week.

How are you supposed to get started? When most people decide that they are going to exercise, they tell themselves that they are going to work out for an hour per day five to seven days per week.

The first day, they jump right in, exercise until they can't move and feel great about it. Then the next day comes, muscles are sore and it becomes harder. By about day three, most people just give up. The reason behind this is because you cannot make huge changes like this and expect them to stick.

Begin small, just in the same way that you took small steps in changing your diet, you will take small steps to change your exercise habits. Begin with 10 minutes of exercise each day, after all, everyone can find 10 minutes per day to exercise and the biggest excuse for not exercising is the lack of time.

After 10 minutes becomes easy for you, add another 5 minutes, exercising 15 minutes per day. Continue to do this until you have worked up to an hour per day.

You also need to remember that you don't have to exercise an hour straight. Exercising 4 times per day for 15 minutes is going to have the same effect on your body as exercising for 1 hour would.

Now it is time to talk about the different types of exercises. Most people will want to begin with aerobic exercises. Aerobic exercise is also known as a cardio workout and is basically any exercise that increases the heart rate as well as the breathing rate. A few examples of aerobic exercises are, dancing, swimming, jogging, biking, and kick boxing. However, there are many day to day activities that can be turned into a cardio workout. For example, mowing the lawn with a push mower, going for a walk after dinner or playing ball with the kids in the yard.

Remember, your cardio workout does not have to be something that you hate, in fact, it should be something that you enjoy otherwise, you are not going to continue to do it.

It is very easy to take cardio too far and it is important that you do not do this. If you have set a goal to do cardio for 30 minutes per day, do that, but don't push yourself to do more. If you find that your body has not recovered completely by the time that you are working out the next day, cut back on the amount of time that you are working out. You should never work so hard that your body does not have time to recover in between workouts.

You should also vary your cardio workouts. While I love sitting on my stationary bike and spinning away, I know that there are muscles in my body that are not getting worked out. It is for that reason that we spend time dancing or playing outside each day, ensuring that not one single muscle group gets over worked but that all of them get the exercise they need. The great thing about cardio exercise is that it is going to boost your metabolism for 24 hours after you finish working out and we have already talked about how a boost in metabolism will help you to lose weight.

The next type of exercise is strength training. When most people think about strength training, they think about a huge muscular man standing in the gym deadlifting 500 pounds. This does not have to be the case. The truth is that you do not have to join a gym, you do not have to bulk up and you do not have to own a set of weights in order to strength train.

There are hundreds of strength training exercises that you can do without any weights and by only using your own body as resistance. Strength training is important when you are losing weight because most of the time, your body is going to use your muscles for energy instead of the stored fat which means you will lose muscle mass. When muscle mass is lost, the metabolic rate drops.

However, when you strength train, your body is able to burn the fat without attacking your muscles first.

Strength training takes longer for your body to recover from than a cardio workout which means that your metabolism is boosted for 36 hours after your workout. Studies have also shown that for every 1 pound of muscle that you gain, your resting metabolic rate goes up between 30 and 50 calories! This means you burn more calories each day!

The key is to ensure that you are not pushing yourself too hard. Just like with cardio workouts, you want to allow your body to rest in between workouts and you want it to be completely recovered before you begin your next workout. This is why you will often see strength trainers focus on one area of their body a day, for example, leg day, arm day and so forth. This allows each area of the body to completely recover while the other areas of the body are being worked out.

The third type of exercise is balance exercises. Balance exercise is not only going to help build muscle but it is also going to help you when you are taking part in your other workouts. Balance exercise helps you to lose weight because it strengthens the muscles and it can be done anywhere and at any time. One balance exercise is walking heel to toe for 20 steps, or standing on one foot and holding for 10 seconds before switching to the next. This type of exercise is not strenuous and it should be practiced every single day.

The fourth and final type of exercise is stretching exercises. These will not only ensure that you are not injured while you are taking part in cardio or strength training, but they will help to strengthen the muscles and can be used to reduce stress. As we have already talked about several times in this book stress has a huge impact on weight loss and weight gain.

These are the four types of exercise and ideally you should be taking part in each one each day. By taking part in all four types of exercise, you will boost your metabolism, increase your muscle mass, reduce your chances of becoming injured and you

will burn calories faster than you can imagine
which means that the pounds will shed off of you.

Chapter 5- Tips to Promote Weight Loss Without Dieting

No one wants to be stuck on a diet for the rest of their lives and no one wants to feel as if there is no hope when it comes to weight loss. In this chapter, I want to talk to you about how you can lose weight without dieting.

Before we begin that, however, I do want to talk a little bit about the foods that you eat. The fact is, that you cannot continue to fill your body with processed foods and expect for it to function properly. This is why I talked about the foods that you should eat for weight loss. This should not be looked at as a diet, but instead is should be looked at as a change you will make in your life so that you can be your happiest and healthiest self.

1. Plan your meals and schedule them. It is very important that you know what you are going to eat and when you are going to eat it. The reason for this is that if you do not know you will have a snack at 9 am and that it is going to be an apple with nut butter,

one of two things will happen. The first is that you will find yourself grazing on food, not really paying attention to what you are eating and the second is that without knowing what you are going to eat, chances are that you are just going to grab something easy for example, a bag of chips.

2. Sleep more. I talked a bit about sleep earlier in this book, but studies have shown that those who sleep at least 8 hours per night weight about 14 pounds less than those who are not getting enough sleep. Your body needs this time to recover from the stress that is put on it during the day and if it is not allowed enough time to recover, the metabolism slows causing you to pack on the pounds.

3. If you serve more vegetables, you are going to eat more vegetables, and if you purchase more vegetables, you will eat more vegetables. Instead of serving fattening sides with your dinner tonight serve sides of vegetables and watch how easy it really is to get the servings you need each day. If

you do not have vegetables in your refrigerator, how can you expect to lose weight and get healthy? When you go shopping, stick to the outside edges of the store, it is usually in the center that the processed junk is found.

4. Eat broth based soup every day. Eating broth based soup is going to allow you to eat your fill while ingesting fewer calories. Not only is it going to help you reduce the amount of calories that you are eating but it is going to ensure you are eating fresh vegetables and it will help you learn how to cook with them as well.

5. Stop eating the sugar filled foods that are made out of white flour and opt for whole grain alternatives. There are so many choices available today and not only is this going to reduce the number of calories that you are eating each day, but it is also going to keep you fuller longer which means a lot less snacking.

6. Get those skinny clothes out, pick out your favorite outfit and hang it where you can

see it every single day. This will be your reminder of what your goals are and it will push you that much further to reach them. If you don't have skinny clothes, head on over to the thrift shop and pick up an adorable outfit that you love and want to fit into. Use this to push you toward your goals.

7. Choose healthy alternatives. Everyone loves pizza, for example, but you don't have to have a slice of pizza with 10 pounds of meat on it. Instead, choose healthier toppings such as peppers, mushrooms, onions or olives and of course go with a whole grain crust.

8. Pay attention to sugar. Sugar that is hidden in the foods that we eat is the real reason that people gain weight. You should only eat about 100 calories worth of sugar each day. Of course, this is refined sugar that is added to your food, not sugar that naturally occurs in fruits and vegetables. Take a walk over to your pantry and look at the amount of sugar that is in the foods you are eating

on a regular basis. Most people are completely unaware of the amount of sugar they are eating and this is why they struggle to lose weight. Did you know that even in reduced calorie versions of foods, the amount of sugar stays the same? This is why you can't depend on these 'diet' foods to help you lose weight.

9. Limit the amount of alcohol you are ingesting. Alcohol provides no nutritional value and is packed full of calories and sugar. If you are out and the occasion calls for a drink, have one, but don't follow it up with another, choose sparkling water instead. Not only does alcohol contain more calories per gram than any other food, but it can also make you completely forget about your diet causing you to inhale an entire bowl of chips in one sitting.

10. Become more mindful. So many of us are focused on other things besides what we are doing right now or what is going on in the moment. We have our meals in front of the television and before we know it, we

have inhaled everything that was on our plate and we are still not satisfied. The reason for this is because our attention is not on the food that we are eating, but on what is going on around us. Start having dinner at the table, focus on what you are eating, how it tastes and enjoy it. This way you will feel satisfied when you have finished your plate.

11. Start eating at home. We are all guilty of it at one time or another. We get too busy; we end up grabbing food on the way home or ordering out simply because we are too tired to cook. However, this is not going to help you lose weight and it is not going to help you be healthy. Quite the contrary. It is understandable that not everyone likes to cook and not everyone is good at it. However, if you want to lose weight, you are going to have to learn. Of course there are going to be a few meals that are going to be hard to swallow, but in time you will be cooking like a chef. When you cook at home, you provide yourself and your family

with healthy foods that are not full of preservatives, you know what is going into the food that you eat.

12. Watch for the eating pause. This is something that most people will do without even realizing it. When a person is eating, there will come a point when they place the silverware on their plate and pause for a moment before picking it back up again. Become aware of this pause, watch for it and when it happens, don't pick the silverware back up again, but instead, clear your plate and move on to something else. This pause signifies that your body is done and does not need any more food.

13. Start chewing gum. When you know that you are at risk from an attack from cravings, pop a piece of strong mint flavored gum in your mouth and watch those cravings pass on by. This is a great way to get your mind off of desert after you have had dinner or off of the cake in the fridge at work.

14. Use smaller plates. The dinner plate is quite large, and it can hold a lot of food. This

really is far too much for the average person to be eating at one sitting. Instead, choose to place your dinner on a salad plate. You will find that you are eating a lot less and that there is no need to go back for seconds. By reducing the size of your plate, you will be reducing your meals by about 100 calories each which means you can lose about 20 pounds per year if not more simply by reducing the size of your plate.

15. Learn about portion size. Something has happened to the sizes of portions people are eating in the United States. As waists grow bigger it seems that portion sizes are as well, however, that is not the case. Portion sizes have always remained the same, it is the number of portions that people are eating that is increasing. Take some time to learn about a serving size, and only eat a serving size instead of eating two or three.

16. Eat meatless meals more often. I will be honest with you. I was the type of person that thought I would die if I did not have

meat with my dinner every night. However, what I quickly learned was that I preferred those light meatless meals to the heavy meals I had been eating. It is so easy to go meatless once or twice a week and you can reduce your calorie intake by about 400 calories per week if not more, it all depends on the amount of meat you were eating before.

17. Push yourself to do just a little more. There are so many activities that you can do to just burn 100 extra calories a day. For example, cleaning the house for 1 hour or mowing the lawn for 20 minutes, or even walking a mile. By burning 100 extra calories a day, you can lose as much as 10 pounds in just 1 year.

18. Reward yourself, just not with food. If you have kicked the soda habit, reward yourself. Do your nails, watch your favorite television show or even buy yourself a new purse with the money you saved on soda. Give yourself something even if it is just an hour alone in

a hot bubble bath, being kind to yourself and rewarding yourself for a job well done.

19. Use the red, orange and green rule. Whenever you eat, you need to make sure that there are foods on your plate of each color. This will ensure that you're getting the healthy vegetables that you need each day. Not only this, but it will ensure that there is no room on your plate for unhealthy junk.

20.   Drink more water. Most people confuse the feeling of thirst with the feeling of hunger, even when they have just had a meal. Instead of grabbing a snack, grab a large glass of water, if you're still hungry afterwards, go ahead and have a snack. You should also drink water as soon as you wake up in the morning in order to boost your metabolism and drink a glass before each meal to ensure you do not over eat.

Losing weight does not have to be complicated, in fact, it can be quite easy if you have the right information. This book gives you that information.

You don't have to go through the rest of your life on yo-yo diets. You don't have to feel bad about not being able to lose weight in the past because you did not have the right information.

Now you have the information, you know that by making small changes in your life, you can start seeing huge results.

Chapter 6- Common Challenges of Weight Loss Tricks

While I discussed many different weight loss tricks in the previous chapter. I want to spend some time in this chapter talking about the challenges that you might face when using these tricks as well as how you can overcome them. There are many tips that I gave you in the previous chapter that are not going to present you with any challenges so they will not all be covered in this chapter. However, I do want to cover the few that could present you with a challenge.

1. When you plan your meals, you have to take into account that life happens. This is something that many diets do not take into account and this often leads to failure. When you know that you are going to be late coming home from work, you can put a meal in the crockpot so that it is ready for you. If you have a hard time finding time to cook during the week, consider using what

is called freezer meals. These are simply home cooked meals that you have prepared ahead of time and are convenient just like prepackaged foods. Always take a snack with you, no matter where you are going. You never know when you are going to get stuck in traffic and see those McDonald arches calling out to you.

2. Sleeping more can seem quite difficult for some people. We are all very busy and there is so much that we have to get done in our days that we often cut back on the amount of time that we are sleeping just to get it done. However, studies show that you are in fact not getting as much done as you think that you are and in fact are halting your productivity by sleeping less. Create a schedule, placing everything that you need to do on it, often times this will allow you to see just how much time is being wasted during your day and it will allow you to find those 8 hours to sleep.

3. Serving more vegetables can become quite difficult, especially if you are not used to

eating vegetables. This is because you will quickly become bored with the same vegetables and all of your meals will tend to be alike. Instead of getting stuck eating the same vegetables every day, expand your palette and try a new vegetable each week. Look online for different ways to prepare your vegetables, ensuring that you are not eating the same ole thing every day.

4. Eating broth based soup is a great way for you to lose weight, however, most people do not want to eat it every day and most people do not want to make it every day. In order to avoid making soup every day, I suggest that you make a large pot on the weekend and separate it out into freezer bags. This will allow you to thaw the soup out on the days that you want to eat it and it will also save time. However, no matter how often you choose to eat broth based soup, you need to eat a variety of foods.

5. When it comes to cutting back on sugar filled foods, you are going to face several challenges. The main one is going to be

cravings. You see, when you eat sugar, it has the same effect on your brain as cocaine. It is safe to say that when you stop eating sugar, your brain reacts the same way as a cocaine addict's brain would react if they were unable to access their drug. This means that you will get weak, often times people feel lightheaded or sick to their stomach and can even get shaky. Not to mention the intense cravings that someone who is quitting sugar has to go through. The way for you to prepare for this is to understand that it is going to happen. Make sure that no matter how bad the cravings get, that you will not give in because it will only make the sugar withdrawals last longer. Remind yourself that this will only last a few days and it will be out of your system, once this happens, don't pick the sugar habit up again.

6. Getting skinny clothes out does not work for some people and if you are one of those people, that is perfectly fine. Some people become discouraged by looking at skinny

clothes and if that is you, simply skip this
tip.

7. When you choose healthy alternatives to
the foods that you are used to eating, you
may find that you feel a bit deprived. If that
is the case, you have to know how to get
around it. You should never feel deprived
while you are eating a healthy diet so if for
example you love meat on your pizza, go
ahead and have meat but top it off with
tons of veggies.

8. It is difficult to eat at home all of the time,
after all, we do have lives. This means that
we have to find a way around eating high
fat foods that are served at restaurants,
parties and other get together. When you
visit a restaurant, don't feel as if you have
to order off of the menu. There is nothing
wrong with ordering a grilled chicken
breast, side salad with lemon juice and oil
with a baked sweet potato. The chef will be
more than happy to make whatever you
want and it does not have to be full of fat
and calories. If you are having a get

together, be the person that is responsible and brings something that you can eat. You have to remember; you are not obligated to eat what is presented to you if you do not feel it is healthy enough. However, you need to remember, everything in moderation. So while you should not eat barbeque burgers every weekend once or twice a summer will be just fine.

The rest of the tricks that I talked about in the previous chapter should not present you with any challenges. However, if you think that a habit or a tip is going to cause challenges for you, it is important for you to sit down and think about how you should react to that challenge before it ever happens. This should be done when you think about the events that are happening in your life as well. For example, a night out with the girls could present many challenges such as overeating and consuming alcohol, completely derailing all of your efforts. While you do deserve a girls' night out, you want to have a plan in place, ensuring that all of the work that you have done thus far was not in vain.

Conclusion:

You don't have to diet any longer. By changing what you eat, adding healthy fruits, vegetables, legumes, whole grains and meats to your diet, you can lose the weight that has plagued you for so long.

Changing the way that you eat is not a stand-alone remedy for losing weight but it must be accompanied by exercise and hydration as well.

In this book, you have learned everything that you need to know to make weight loss finally work for you, ensuring that you see the results you so desire. Now all that is left for you to do is start taking action.

It is your time. Time for you to finally live the life you have always wanted to live and look how you have always wanted to look.

Weight Loss Tricks: Tips to Escape the Dieting Trap;
No Miracles, Just Facts

Copyright ©2016 by CHARLES BENSON

All rights reserved. No part of this book may be
reproduced or transmitted in any form or by any
means without written permission from the author.

www.ingramcontent.com/pod-product-compliance
Lightning Source LLC
Chambersburg PA
CBHW071121280526
45787CB00003B/1120